Introduction

Organisms related contaminations and sicknesses have been a developing issue all around the world because of their high therapy cost, and as a rule, it is underdiagnosed. Perhaps the most widely recognized contamination particularly to ladies is what we call Candidiasis or Yeast Infection. It is extremely pervasive that the absolute expense of hospitalization for it in the United States arrived at a gauge of $1.4 billion in 2017.[1]

That astounding number was taken uniquely in the United States, yet it is a worldwide issue that is influencing around 138 million ladies everywhere, 9 million of whom are ladies from the US. These numbers back up past exploration that 75% of the female populace experience the ill effects of this condition and around 6% of them manage recurrence.[2]

Everyone has specific measures of growths inside their bodies and, typically, it doesn't actually hurt. Be that as it may, because of different variables, the equilibrium might be tipped and those changes will achieve conditions like yeast disease. It is ordinarily a medical condition of females, however guys can likewise procure it.

Some meds are successful in treating yeast contaminations. Some of them are accessible and sold as over-the-counter meds in drug stores, however a way of life change will likewise help hugely in dealing with this condition.

For instance, our eating regimen can influence our vulnerability to these parasitic contaminations, thus our odds of procuring such conditions can be limited just by arranging our suppers carefully.

We really want to remember that organisms can endure even in troublesome conditions, and generally, they are simply sitting tight for the valuable chance to fill in numbers and begin creating some issues. Having said that, realizing that these microorganisms are inside our bodies, we have the obligation to at minimum attempt to secure ourselves. This we can do with the assistance of a well-arranged eating routine plan.

If you are searching for an educational bit by bit guide in after an enemy of yeast diet, continue to peruse this guide.

Here's an outline of what you will find in this guide:

- What yeast contamination is for women
- How to forestall and treat yeast infection
- The sorts of food you ought to consume and remain from

- 2-week bit by bit manual for follow an enemy of yeast diet
- Sample plans that can assist you with this specific diet

Chapter 1: What You Need to Know About Yeast Infection

What is a yeast infection?
It is a condition when Candida albicans, a kind of growth that is typically present in our body, duplicates in significant sums to the point of causing wellbeing problems.

Yeast disease is otherwise called candidiasis. It very well may be found in explicit region of the body like the mouth, intestinal system, throat, and vagina. In ladies, the vaginal region is the most widely recognized site of disease, henceforth why this condition is likewise alluded to as vaginal candidiasis, vulvovaginal candidiasis, and candida vaginitis. [3]

What are the causes of yeast infection in women?
We know at this point that candida is inside our bodies from the beginning. The inquiry triggers these parasites into multiplying?

- Hormones. Females who are taking conception prevention pills are in danger of getting yeast diseases because of the progressions yet to be determined occurring in their regenerative framework. This is additionally pertinent to breastfeeding mothers and ladies who are pregnant.

- Vaginal showers and douches. Utilizing these items isn't fitting as these too can cause lopsided characteristics in ladies' vagina. [4]

- Antibiotics. Ladies who have different contaminations might be endorsed anti-toxins to deal with their conditions, yet these meds may likewise eliminate the great microscopic organisms dwelling in vaginas.

- Uncontrolled diabetes. On the off chance that not oversaw accurately, diabetic patients might have significant degrees of sugar in their pee, and this sugar will take care of Candida albicans, making them become further and multiply.

- Compromised safe framework. Different sicknesses that can cause the debilitating of the safe framework, similar to HIV and AIDS, can likewise make the vagina helpless against yeast infection.

What are the signs and symptoms of vaginal yeast infection?

- Swelling and redness in the vulva and vaginal area
- Burning sensation in the vagina particularly while peeing and during

intercourse

- Irritation and irritation in the vagina and vulva
- Rashes in the vaginal area
- Pain and touchiness of the vagina
- Unusual release that is either watery or white and thick like house cheese

How is yeast infection diagnosed?
Unlike different growths related diseases and ailments, yeast contamination is very simple to analyze. Your physician will interview you and ask questions about your medical history, such as if you had yeast infections before and if you ever had sexually transmitted infections in the past.

Next, your doctor should analyze you further, particularly in the pelvic region, including your vaginal region. Yeast disease in the vagina generally gives indications remotely, so your PCP will actually want to distinguish it clinically during the exam.

Depending on the clinical examination, the doctor might order some lab tests to be done with cells gathered from your vagina to be certain of their diagnosis. It is important to note though that most of the time, samples are only taken from those females who have recurring infections.[5]

When to see your doctor?
Whether you are thinking you have a yeast contamination or you had it previously, it is ideal to be checked by your doctor or gynecologist when:

- You suspect to have it regardless of whether you've never had a yeast contamination before.
- You utilized enemy of contagious meds you purchased over-the-counter yet side effects persist.
- You are beginning to foster different manifestations of this infection.

Chapter 2: Prevention and Treatment for Yeast Infection in Women

How to Prevent Yeast Infection
Just on the grounds that yeast disease is normal in ladies, doesn't mean it can't be forestalled. Coming up next are ways that can assist with forestalling this sort of infection:

- Avoid wearing tight-base apparel like jeans, pantyhose, stockings, and the preferences. All things being equal, wear garments that are free, or on the other hand assuming you should wear tight garments, ensure they are made with normal filaments like material, silk, and cotton.

- Refrain from utilizing scented female items like sterile cushions, tampons, fragrances, and deodorants.
- Limit washing in steaming hot water and drenching for too long.
- Change your wet dress like swimsuits and the preferences when possible.
- Avoid utilizing douches. This will just eliminate the great microbes that guide in warding off parasitic infections.
- In picking oils, go all of the time with the water-based type.
- Refrain from changing female items time and again as this might disturb the vulva and vaginal regions that might prompt yeast infection.
- Do not take anti-microbials on the off chance that not required, particularly when you just have a typical cold and other gentle diseases that don't need such medication.
- Follow a sound and adjusted eating regimen implied for your condition.
- Lessen utilization of desserts as sugar fills in as nourishment for candida.
- Shower after oral sex and sexual intercourse.
- Thoroughly dry the genital region after washing or showering and prior to wearing clothing and clothing.
- Wash underpants utilizing boiling water to kill off any growths that don't ordinarily kick the bucket with simply normal washing.
- Consider taking probiotic enhancements to support your lactobacillus count that assists with fending off Candida albicans.[6]

How to Treat Yeast Infection

Depending on your particular case, your doctor will either expose you to a short or long haul treatment. This will not set in stone by how often you get the disease and its severity.

For the novices and those ladies who just display gentle to direct indications, the specialists typically recommend antifungal meds that can be purchased over-the-counter or by remedy. These are ordinarily in the types of suppositories, skin creams, or balms, or even tablets to be taken for a couple of days up to a week.

For women who frequently experience yeast infections and show severe and more complicated symptoms, the doctors will subject them to a longer treatment plan. Antifungal medications prescribed are usually taken daily for up to 2 weeks and weekly for the next 6 months.[7]

Additionally, women who have frequent infections may be subjected to test for HIV or AIDS and other necessary tests to find out if there is an underlying cause of yeast infection that was not diagnosed before. Proper treatment of the root cause of the problem will prevent a recurrence.[8]

Lastly, the board of yeast disease doesn't just include the one contaminated yet additionally their accomplices, particularly assuming they are physically dynamic. This case is generally normal with ladies who have incessant diseases regardless of not having foundational conditions like diabetes thus. They should utilize insurance to stop the pattern of repeating disease until they are both treated.[9]

Alternative Medicine and Home Remedies for Yeast Infection

As existing apart from everything else, there are no dependable elective meds accessible in the market to treat yeast contamination, however there are medicines that might assist with lightening the side effects. Best to counsel first with your primary care physician to get legitimate treatment.

There are a few home cures known to assist with overseeing yeast diseases. Notwithstanding, it isn't demonstrated to be pretty much as powerful as real medicines
delivered exclusively to treat this condition. It's additionally energetically prescribed to counsel first with your wellbeing proficient when wanting to utilize any of these home remedies.

Coming up next are the most widely recognized home solutions for yeast infection:

- Boric acid. This contains antiseptic properties that can help stop the overgrowth of yeast if used as a vaginal suppository. However, because of its potency, it is not advised to be used as the first line of treatment. Instead, go for a milder option.[10]

- Vitamin C. This nutrient is known to assist with supporting the resistant framework. By taking the suggested every day portion, the odds of recuperating from yeast contamination will be considerably higher.

- Tea tree oil. There are claims that vaginal suppositories that contain this rejuvenating ointment can assist with killing Candida albicans with their antifungal properties. [11]

- Hydrogen peroxide. Although this has not been specifically used on strains of yeast in vaginal infections in studies, this strong antiseptic can kill the yeast. Precaution must be taken if it will be applied to the vagina, and it should be diluted to avoid causing irritations.[12]
- Oreganum oil. This is otherwise called oregano oil and has been found powerful in repressing the development of Candida albicans because of its antifungal properties. [13]

- Probiotic supplements. Beside food and beverages, probiotics currently come as pills and powders. These will assist with supporting your security from yeast and are normally embedded into the vagina as suppositories.

Chapter 3: Identify Your Limits

There are discusses in regards to the adequacy and need of an enemy of yeast diet. Certain individuals say that after a severe eating routine like this isn't demonstrated to stop the abundance of Candida albicans, however realizing what kinds of food to eat and stay away from can help in fundamentally resetting your body's microbiome and further developing stomach health.[14]

What types of food should you eat?
This diet is centered around getting better and slender proteins, great fats, and green verdant vegetables. Here are some examples:

- Avocado is a decent wellspring of solid fats
- Non-bland and cruciferous vegetables like zucchini, asparagus, cabbage, broccoli, Brussels sprout, and cauliflower
- Green verdant vegetables like lettuce, spinach, and kale
- Healthy wellsprings of protein, for example, eggs, chicken and turkey bosoms, and grass-took care of beef
- Tree nuts like almonds, macadamia, and walnuts
- Seeds like flaxseed, chia seeds, and hemp seeds
- Aromatics like ginger, garlic, shallots, and onions
- Herbs and flavors like basil, cilantro, oregano, cumin, and turmeric
- Fruits that have low sugar content like berries and tomatoes
- Some restricted dairy items like margarine and ghee
- Natural yogurt (most ideally with negligible sugar content)
- Olive and coconut oil
- Dark chocolate
- Green tea

Probiotic beverages and food like yogurt can assist with upsetting the development of yeast, so it is great to fuse them into your eating routine. Despite the fact that yogurt is aged, it is permitted in this eating routine because of the great number of solid microorganisms it contains that will help fend off Candida albicans. Having said that, devouring yogurt should in any case be controlled and should not surpass the limits.

What types of food should you avoid?

The food limitations in this diet are for the most part towards, however not restricted to, food sources with handled or refined sugar and flour. Here are some of them:

- Sweet organic products like mangoes, bananas, and grapes
- Sugar and syrups, particularly high fructose corn syrup
- Dairy items like milk and cheese
- Starchy vegetables and root crops like carrots and potatoes
- Fermented cocktails like brew, juices, wines, and champagne
- Dried meats like relieved bacon, hams, wieners, and hotdogs
- Dried or canned organic products like peaches, cranberries, raisins, and prunes
- Mushrooms
- Sweet treats like cakes, frozen yogurt, pies, brownies, etc.
- Foods that are made of flour like cakes, bread, pizza, pasta, bagels, and the likes
- Pistachios and peanuts

It is additionally prudent to restrict yourself from eating matured food sources like kimchi, pickles, soy sauce, vinegar, and aged beverages like fermented tea. These are alright to eat and drink in the end however not while you are as yet encountering a yeast infection.

Chapter 4: How to Start Your Diet Plan

You definitely know the kinds of food you can eat and those that you ought to keep away from. You can now begin making your eating regimen arrangements, yet the inquiry is, the way do you start?

In this part and the following, you will see a bit by bit guide that will assist you with beginning your enemy of yeast diet.

WEEK 1: Make a Weekly Meal Plan

Following a severe eating routine, like this one, can be a little problem. Dissimilar to previously, you can't simply look at your storage space and set up whatever is in there to make your suppers since you presently have food restrictions.

A method for taking care of this issue is by making a dinner arrangement each week with the goal that you will know precisely what fixings to purchase during your staple excursions. By doing this, you additionally will not need to ponder what food to eat during your meals.

Think pretty much every one of the dinners you like, write them all down, and from those, eliminate the ones that contain fixings that you really want to stay away from. With the suppers that you have left on your rundown, convey them to your week after week feast spread as one or the other breakfast, lunch, or supper. Assuming there are unfilled spots remaining, fill them with other quality dinners that you can in any case join into this diet.

Here is an example of a 7-day supper intend to assist you with getting started:

DAY	BREAKFAST	LUNCH	DINNER
1	Cinnamon Quinoa Bowl	Zucchini Celery Soup	Roast Chicken and Asparagus
2	Tofu Scramble	Roasted Tomato Soup	Lemon Garlic Baked Salmon
3	Vegan scones with berries	Green Gazpacho	Coconut Artichoke Soup
4	Chickpea and Onion Omelette	Garlic Buttered Shrimps	Watermelon Tomato Salad
5	Tomato Frittatas with Kale and Dill	Baked Flounder	Mixed Berries and Kale Salad
6	Broccoli Quinoa Cakes	White Bean Stew	Roast Beef and Cauliflower Rice
7	Chickpea Scramble with Zucchini	French Onion Soup	Salmon Salad

Helpful Tip: Condition Your Body

Our eating regimen is essential for our way of life, and an unexpected change in that can be testing, so it is ideal to set up your psyche and body before the entire eating routine makeover starts.

Try to detoxify your framework to assist your body with acclimating to the new eating regimen. You can drink detox teas as these will assist with ousting poisons from the body and permit better retention of supplements when you authoritatively start this new journey.

Chapter 5: How to Follow an Anti-Yeast Diet

Now that you have figured out a week after week supper plan, the time has come to get everything rolling on this new journey.

WEEK 2: Implementation

Part of your street to recuperation from yeast disease doesn't simply end in dinner arranging. You want to execute it adequately and at last completely fuse it into your way of life particularly assuming you are encountering the disease over and over.

Step 1: Gather and Prepare Your Ingredients

It is essential that you get every one of the required elements for this supper plan that you made, ideally week by week too. Try to get them as new as could really be expected and just from stores that are trusted to sell great quality and clean produce.

Yeast disease can likewise make you defenseless to different growths related contaminations thus, you really want to examine your fixings cautiously. Clean the entirety of your fixings completely and eliminate anything that looks filthy and stained as these might be polluted with molds.

Step 2: Always Check the Labels

Sometimes we can't try not to purchase pre-stuffed food varieties and canned products henceforth the should be extremely careful in purchasing our ingredients.

Some food sources have stowed away sugars that we may not know about, and on the grounds that sugar is something that ought to be wiped out in an enemy of yeast diet, you should consistently check the names and ensure that you won't devour something not really great for your condition.

Step 3: Start Prepping Your Meals

Not all dinners from your eating routine arrangement should be cooked newly without fail. Subsequently, saving you some time in setting up these suppers ahead. An illustration of a food that you can plan from the get-go in the week is your servings of mixed greens. You can cleave every one of your greens and vegetables, put them in hermetically sealed compartments, and spot them in the refrigerator since the vast majority of these fixings need not be cooked.

For different suppers that require cooking, you can divide them early and assemble them in various holders. At the point when the time has come to make them, you can simply remove them from the ice chest, and you will have all that you really want for every particular meal.

Being coordinated will save you time and will assist with keeping away from

startling problems. Stage 4: Stay Hydrated

We have been instructed 100% concerning the time to drink no less than 8 glasses of water day by day; nonetheless, a few examinations recommend that the day by day measure of water required by every individual shifts. [15]

Regardless, it is as yet a well established reality that we really want to drink sufficient water every day to remain solid. Considering that reality, water actually assumes a major part in after an enemy of yeast diet.

Drinking bunches of water will cause you to pee all the more frequently and in doing as such, will help flush out more poisons out of your body. It will likewise assist your stomach with remaining solid and hold onto yeast overgrowth.

Additionally, expanding your water admission can likewise assist you with feeling full, which will support controlling your cravings.

Step 4: Control Your Cravings

Dairy items are only a couple of the things you really want to keep away from in after this eating regimen, however let's be honest, cheddar is a tasty food, and staying away from it will be a test. Anyway, how would you be able to treat you are having significant longings? The response is by replacement. You will most likely be unable to eat all that you used to eat, however you can eat substitutes when the desires are solid. Here are a few food varieties that you can eat as replacements:

- If you are feeling the loss of your morning toasts severely, you can utilize tortillas rather as these don't contain yeast.
- When longing for peanuts or pistachios, you can eat tree nuts rather like almonds, macadamia, and walnuts.
- Missing peanut butter? Attempt almond butter.
- If you are in the state of mind for some, potato chips, take a stab at

making seared garlic chips or fresh kale chips.

Following this diet might represent a test, however with a great deal of choices accessible for you, this ought to have the option to propel you to continue to give a shot to prevail with this diet.

Chapter 6: Sample Recipes

Here are a few example plans that you can consolidate into your enemy of yeast diet:

Roasted Veggies

Ingredients:

- ✔ 1/2 lb. turnips
- ✔ 1/2 lb. carrots
- ✔ 1/2 lb. parsnips
- ✔ 2 shallots, peeled
- ✔ 1/4 tsp. ground dark pepper
- ✔ 1 tbsps. extra-virgin olive oil
- ✔ 6 cloves garlic
- ✔ 3/4 tsp. fit salt
- ✔ 2 tbsp. new rosemary needles

Instructions:

1. First, cut vegetables into reduced down pieces.
2. Set the stove to 400°F.
3. Mix every one of the fixings in a baking dish.
4. Roast the vegetables for 25 minutes until brown and tender.
5. Toss and meal again for 20-25 minutes.
6. Serve and appreciate while hot.

Spinach and Watercress Salad

Ingredients:

- ✔ 1 cup watercress, washed with stems removed
- ✔ 3 cups child spinach, washed with stems removed
- ✔ 1 medium cut avocado
- ✔ 1/4 cup avocado oil
- ✔ 1/8 cup lemon juice
- ✔ a touch of salt

Instructions:

1. Pat dry the spinach and watercress. Eliminate the stem and separate the leaves.

2. On an enormous serving plate, consolidate the leaves of the watercress and the spinach.
3. Cut the avocado in half then, at that point, eliminate the pit. Strip the skin off from each side.
4. Slice the avocadoes into dainty strips. Set aside.
5. Prepare the dressing by joining avocado oil and lemon juice.
6. Arrange the avocado strips on top of the watercress and spinach.
7. Season with salt and pepper.
8. Drizzle with the dressing before serving.

Mixed Vegetable Roast with Lemon Zest

Ingredients:

- ✔ 1-1/2 cups broccoli florets
- ✔ 1-1/2 cups cauliflower florets
- ✔ 3/4 cup red ringer pepper, diced
- ✔ 3/4 cup zucchini, diced
- ✔ 2 daintily cut cloves of garlic
- ✔ 2 tsp. lemon zest
- ✔ 1 tbsp. olive oil
- ✔ A spot of salt
- ✔ 1 tsp. dried and squashed

oregano Instructions:

1. Preheat the broiler, set to 425°F.
2. Combine garlic and the two florets in a baking container. Shower oil over the vegetables and sprinkle with salt and oregano; mix enough to cover. Broil for 10 minutes.
3. Add zucchini and ringer pepper to the remainder of the blend in the container; throw to combine.
4. Continue simmering until the pieces are delicately seared and are fresh tender.
5. Before serving, sprinkle lemon zing over the vegetables and toss.
6. Enjoy while hot.

Salmon and Asparagus

Ingredients:

- ✔ 2 salmon fillets
- ✔ 14 ounces youthful potatoes
- ✔ 8 asparagus lances, managed and halved
- ✔ 2 small bunches cherry tomatoes
- ✔ 1 small bunch basil leaves
- ✔ 2 tbsp. extra-virgin olive oil

- ✔ 1 tbsp. balsamic vinegar

Instructions:

1. Heat broiler to 428°F.
2. Arrange potatoes into a baking dish.
3. Drizzle potatoes with extra-virgin olive oil.
4. Roast potatoes until they have become brilliant brown.
5. Place asparagus into the baking dish along with the potatoes.
6. Roast in the stove for 15 minutes.
7. Arrange cherry tomatoes and salmon among the vegetables.
8. Shower with balsamic vinegar and the excess olive oil.
9. Roast until salmon is cooked.
10. Throw in basil leaves prior to moving everything to a serving dish.
11. Serve while hot.

Arugula and Mushroom Salad

Ingredients:

- ✔ 5 oz. arugula washed
- ✔ 1 lb. new mushrooms
- ✔ 1/4 teaspoon shoyu
- ✔ 1/2 red onion
- ✔ 1 tbsp. olive oil
- ✔ 1 tbsp. mirin

To make tofu cheese:

- ✔ 1/8 cup umeboshi vinegar
- ✔ 1/2 firm tofu

Instructions:

1. In a bowl, add the washed tofu. Disintegrate and pour in vinegar.
2. In a different bowl add shoyu, red onions, salt, olive oil, and mirin. Blend to combine.
3. Add in the arugula and throw to consolidate with the dressing.
4. Serve and enjoy.

Seafood Stew

Ingredients:

- ✔ 2 tsp. extra-virgin olive oil
- ✔ 1 cut bulb fennel
- ✔ 2 stems celery, chopped
- ✔ 2 cups white wine

- ✔ 1 tbsp. slashed thyme
- ✔ 1 cup hacked shallots
- ✔ 6 ounces shrimp
- ✔ 6 ounces of ocean scallops
- ✔ 1/4 tsp. salt
- ✔ 1 cup slashed parsley
- ✔ 6 oz. icy char
- ✔ 2-1/2 cups of water

Instructions:

1. Heat a skillet on the most reduced oven setting. Put a modest quantity of oil.
2. Cook the celery, shallots, and fennel for roughly 6 minutes.
3. Pour in the wine, water, and thyme into the singing pan.
4. Wait for 10 minutes and permit it to cook.
5. Once a significant part of the water has vanished, include the leftover fixings, and hang tight for 2 minutes prior to eliminating from the stove.
6. Serve and appreciate immediately.

Tomato Clams

Ingredients:

- ✔ Canola oil cooking spray
- ✔ 1 onion, sliced
- ✔ 1 tsp. minced garlic, or to taste
- ✔ 1/2 tsp salt
- ✔ 3 pounds of shellfishes, in shell, completely scrubbed
- ✔ 1 tsp red pepper flakes
- ✔ 1 cup white wine
- ✔ 1/2 lb. entire grain linguine, cooked by bundle directions
- ✔ 1/2 cup level leaf parsley, chopped
- ✔ 4 cups cherry tomatoes, divided

Instructions:

1. Heat a huge pot with a cover over low heat.
2. Spray with vegetable oil cooking shower and add the onion, garlic, and salt. Cook for 3 minutes, blending constantly.
3. Add the mollusks, red pepper chips, and wine
4. Cover and stew until the shellfishes open, around 7 minutes. Dispose of those shellfishes that don't open.
5. Add the pasta, parsley, and tomatoes. Cover and let stew for 3 extra minutes. Mix and serve immediately.

Baked Flounder

Ingredients:

- ✔ 1 lb. fumble fillet
- ✔ 1 tbsp. extra-virgin olive oil
- ✔ 1/4 tsp. salt
- ✔ Freshly ground dark pepper to taste
- ✔ 1 cup divided red grapes
- ✔ 1 cup hacked and toasted almonds
- ✔ 2 tbsp. finely cleaved parsley
- ✔ 1 tbsp. lemon juice

Instructions:

1. Preheat the broiler to 375°F. Put fish on a sheet plate and season with 1-1/2 tsp. of olive oil, 1/8 tsp of salt, and newly ground dark pepper.
2. In a bowl, consolidate the grapes, almonds, parsley, lemon juice, 1-1/2 tsp. of olive oil, 1/8 tsp of salt, and dark pepper.
3. Place the fish in the stove and heat for 3 minutes, flip the fish, return to the broiler until the fish is simply starting to chip however the middle is as yet clear around 3 minutes. Take care not to overcook
4. Remove from the broiler and serve promptly, finished off with the grape mixture.

Vegan Pesto

Ingredients:

- ✔ 1-1/2 cups new basil
- ✔ 1/3 cup olive oil (or other superior grade and tasty oil)
- ✔ 1 cup pine nuts
- ✔ 5 cloves garlic
- ✔ 1/3 cup nourishing yeast
- ✔ 3/4 teaspoon salt
- ✔ 1/2 teaspoon dark pepper

Instructions:

1. Combine all fixings in a food processor until nuts are ground.
2. Pesto should in any case have surface and not be totally smooth.
3. Add more salt and pepper to taste.

Spinach and Chickpeas

Ingredients:

- ✔ 3 tbsp. additional virgin olive oil
- ✔ 1 onion, meagerly sliced

- ✔ 4 cloves garlic, minced
- ✔ 1 tbsp. ground ginger
- ✔ ½ holder grape tomatoes
- ✔ 1 lemon, zested and newly juiced
- ✔ 1 tsp. squashed red pepper flakes
- ✔ 1 enormous jar of chickpeas
- ✔ 6 cups spinach
- ✔ Sea salt to taste

Instructions:

1. Add additional virgin olive oil to a huge skillet, add onion, and cook until the onion starts to brown.
2. Add garlic, ginger, tomatoes, lemon zing, red pepper chips, and spinach. Cook for around 3 to 4 minutes.
3. Add cooked chickpeas and mix. Add oil if necessary.
4. Serve and enjoy.

Zucchini and Celery Greens Soup

Ingredients:

- ✔ 1/2 cup cooked green lentils
- ✔ 1 parsnip, stripped and finely diced
- ✔ 1 onion, finely diced
- ✔ 2 garlic cloves, crushed
- ✔ 1 green ringer pepper, cut into little cubes
- ✔ 4 asparagus spears
- ✔ 1 little zucchini, sliced
- ✔ 1 little fennel bulb, finely diced
- ✔ 2 celery stems, finely diced
- ✔ 1 little bundle of celery greens or different greens accessible: kale, spinach beet greens
- ✔ 1 lime juice only
- ✔ 2 cups low sodium vegetable broth
- ✔ 1 tsp. chia seeds to garnish
- ✔ Freshly ground dark pepper

Instructions:

1. In a medium pot, fry the onions and garlic for 2 minutes, blending frequently.
2. Add the celery stems, fennel, zucchini, ringer pepper, and parsnip, along with the vegetable broth.
3. Bring to bubble, then, at that point, stew on low hotness for 7 minutes.
4. Add the lentils, asparagus, celery greens, and lime juice. Turn the hotness off.

5. Serve warm, decorated with chia seeds.

Tahini Salmon

Instructions:

- ✔ 1/4 cup tahini
- ✔ 3 tbsp. new lemon juice
- ✔ 1 tsp. pounded garlic
- ✔ 1/4 tsp. salt
- ✔ 1/2 cup finely slashed cilantro
- ✔ 2 tbsp. generally slashed toasted walnuts
- ✔ 2 tbsp. generally slashed toasted almonds
- ✔ 1 tbsp. finely slashed onion
- ✔ 1 tsp. extra-virgin olive oil
- ✔ Pinch of cayenne, or to taste
- ✔ Freshly ground dark pepper to taste
- ✔ 1 lb. wild salmon skin eliminated, new or frozen

Instructions:

1. In a bowl, join the tahini, 2 tbsp. of lemon juice, 3 tbsp. of water, crushed garlic, and 1/8 tsp of salt; set aside
2. In a different bowl, join the cilantro, pecans, almonds, onion, olive oil, cayenne, dark pepper, and 1/8 tsp. of salt.
3. Fill the lower part of a liner with water and carry to a boil.
4. Season fish with 1 tbsp. for lemon juice.
5. Place it on a plate and set it on the highest point of the liner. Cover and cook, taking consideration to eliminate while the fish is as yet pink inside, around 3 to 4 minutes.
6. Remove the fish from the liner, top with the tahini blend, and afterward with the cilantro mixture.
7. Serve warm or at room temperature.

Tomato and Basil Soup

Ingredients:

- ✔ 1 onion
- ✔ 1 clove of garlic
- ✔ 2 tbsp. olive oil
- ✔ 8 cherry tomatoes/3 plant tomatoes
- ✔ 14 oz. can plum tomatoes
- ✔ 1 tsp. dried basil or 5 leaves of new basil
- ✔ 150 ml. water
- ✔ 1 tsp. salt
- ✔ Pepper

Instructions:

1. Chop onion and tomatoes. Finely cut the garlic.
2. Sauté in olive oil onion, tomatoes, garlic, and basil.
3. Add canned tomatoes, salt, and pepper. Cover the container and let it stew for 30 minutes on low heat.
4. Transfer to a blender or food processor and mix until smooth.
5. Serve and enjoy.

Cauliflower and Mushroom Bake

Ingredients:

- ✔ 3 cups cauliflower florets
- ✔ 1 cup new mushroom, chopped
- ✔ 1/2 cup red onion, chopped
- ✔ 1/3 cup green onion, chopped
- ✔ 2 garlic cloves, finely chopped
- ✔ 2 tsp. apple juice vinegar
- ✔ 2 tsp. lemon juice
- ✔ 1/2 tsp. salt
- ✔ 1/4 tsp. pepper
- ✔ 1 tbsp. olive oil

Instructions:

1. Preheat the stove to 350°F. Delicately oil a baking pan.
2. Combine red onion, cauliflower, olive oil, garlic, mushroom, apple juice vinegar, lemon squeeze, salt, and pepper in a bowl. Blend well.
3. Pour the combination into the lubed baking pan.
4. Place inside the stove and heat for 45 minutes. Stir.
5. When vegetables are brilliant brown and delicate, eliminate from the oven.
6. Garnish with green onions. Serve and enjoy.

Conclusion

Yeast contamination on ladies is something that shouldn't be overlooked nor trifled with. It's vital to promptly have your PCP checked for side effects on the off chance that you presume you have this disease. Different medicines are accessible, contingent upon the seriousness and what your primary care physician might recommend to you.

If you are investigating shunning having the contamination, regardless of whether you've never had it or it's a common disease, you can evaluate this enemy of yeast diet. It may not actually tackle the issue, yet it will assist you with monitoring yourself against securing it. Something else, the counter yeast diet plan is likewise helpful for your whole prosperity. Make sure to consistently counsel first with your primary care physician or an authorized dietician prior to evaluating this diet plan.

Thank you again for getting this guide.

If you found this guide supportive, kindly invest in some opportunity to share your contemplations and post an audit. It'd be extraordinarily appreciated!

Thank you and great luck!

www.ingramcontent.com/pod-product-compliance
Lightning Source LLC
LaVergne TN
LVHW041309150826
845673LV00008B/2808

* 9 7 9 8 4 1 8 7 1 2 5 2 3 *